MY FOOD NIGHTMARES
LIVING WITH ARFID

Fernanda do Valle and

Giovana Vasconcellos

UNDERLINE
PUBLISHING

ISBN 978-1-962185-31-8

Copyright text © 2024 Fernanda do Valle
and
Giovana Vasconcellos
Translation Daniel Mantellato

1ª edition, 2024

Published by Underline Publishing LLC
www.underlinepublishing.com

MY FOOD NIGHTMARES
LIVING WITH ARFID

Fernanda do Valle and
Giovana Vasconcellos

To my children, Daniel and Theo, my "bonus kids" Hugo Leonardo, Karinna, Thalita, Jamie, and Elie, and my wife and love of my life, Ilana. Also, to all the families who have trust in my work and my clients who teach and inspire me in my professional growth.

Fernanda

To my daughter, Antonella, my Tonton. She is a fulfillment, an inspiration and an impulse for my personal growth. To my husband, Guilherme, who supports me at all times, and my family, who celebrate and experience all my accomplishments with me. Also, to my clients - believe me, you are the ones who teach me every day - and to my colleagues, who are crucial to my professional growth.

Giovana

CONTENTS

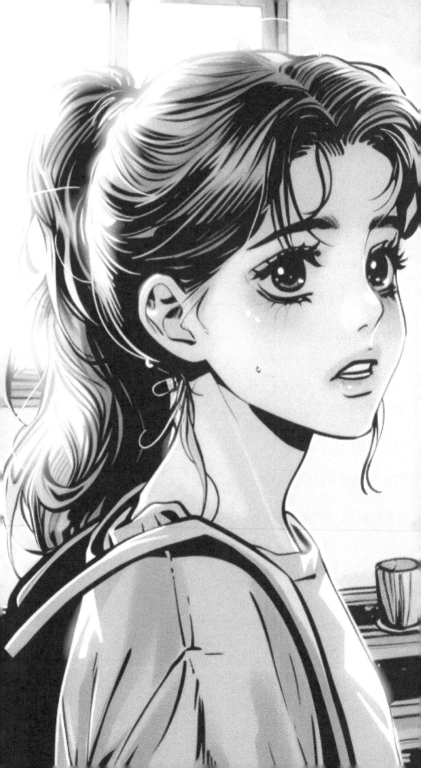

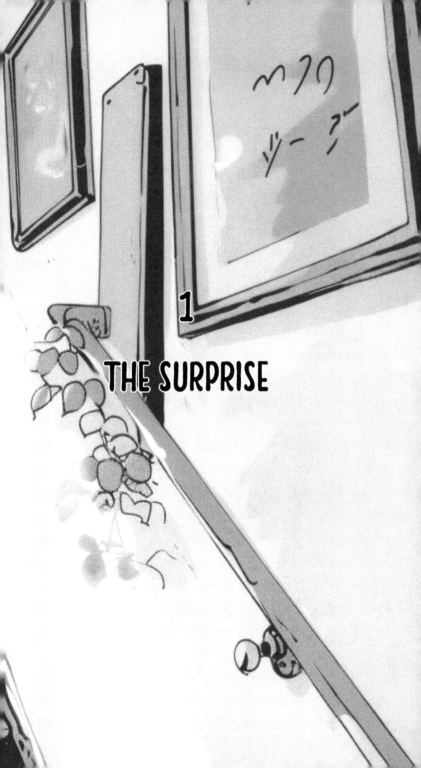

1

THE SURPRISE

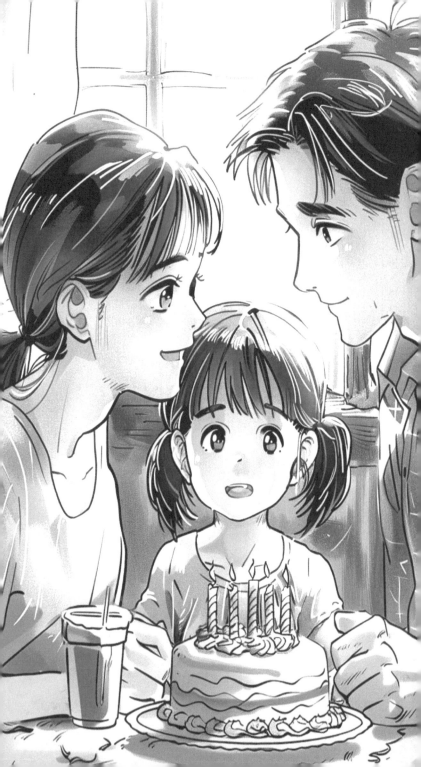

THE SURPRISE

Tonton was known for being a very happy and charismatic young girl who loved to spend time with family and friends. She grew up and developed just like any other girl her age, and she was always complimented by her friends and adults around her for being extremely smart, fun, and creative. She was popular in school and was an A+ student. Everyone liked to play with her.

Her birthday was coming up, and just like any other year, Tonton's mom was planning a wonderful party. This year, however, her birthday was even more special. Tonton would be celebrating her 12th birthday, and her mom would always tell her that turning twelve years old was something magical.

"Tonton, your birthday party will be perfect! Perfect just like you!" Said Tonton's mom several times throughout that year.

The party was scheduled for the 10th of December 2023. The invitations had already been sent out and all of those invited were waiting anxiously for the day to arrive. Two weeks before the party, on a cold and rainy Friday afternoon, Tonton arrives from school and, to her parents' surprise, announces with a firm voice, trying not to cry:

"Mom, dad, I don't want a party... I don't want to celebrate my birthday this year and I don't want to talk about it."

Shocked, her parents could not understand the reason for such a sudden and unexpected request. Tonton always loved her birthdays and would count down the days for her party.

Tonton, no longer holding in her tears, cried a lot and could not organize her thoughts, and as such, could not talk about her feelings.

Her parents were lost. They kept asking her question after question trying to understand what was happening, drowning her with their words.

Tonton once again said she did not want to talk about the matter and ran to her room, which was her safe place when she wanted to be alone. She slammed the door and jumped in bed, covering her head with her blue blanket filled with white unicorns that glowed in the dark. The safe blanket always calmed her down when needed. She stayed there for hours, protecting herself from the outside world, wishing she would never return to her real life.

Her parents remained in the living room, motionless. They looked at each other, not knowing what to do, what to say, and not understanding what caused their daughter's suffering. Even though Tonton had run up to her room and asked to be alone countless times in the past, this was the first time her parents had seen her in that emotional state.

They decided to wait for their daughter to calm down to try to talk to her again.

2
THE CONVERSATION

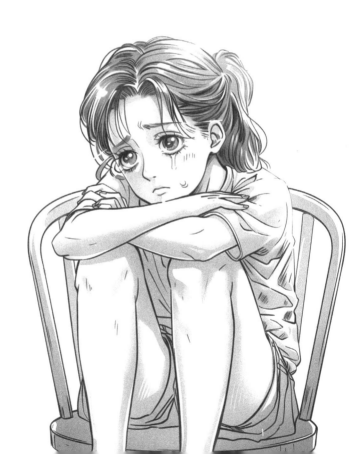

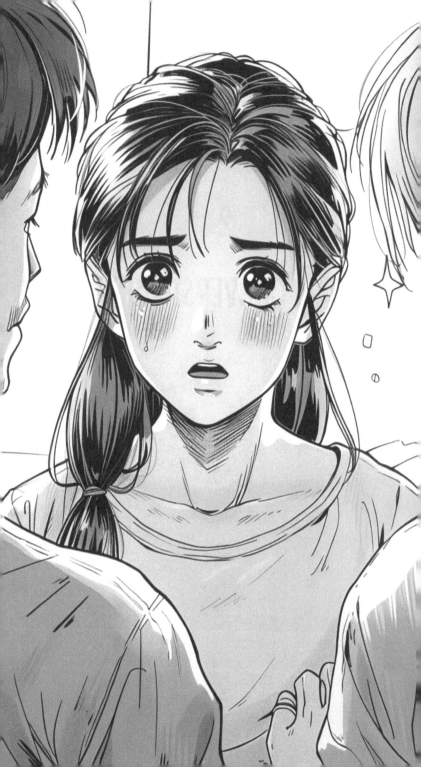

THE CONVERSATION

It was already dark out when Tonton returned to the living room to talk to her parents.

With puffy eyes from all the crying she had done, Tonton said:

"Mom… dad… I think I am prepared to talk about this now. I can't hold this inside me any longer. I am ashamed that I can barely eat anything. In the past, I was able to pretend, but now that I eat even less, I can't hide it anymore."

"For some time now, my friends keep asking me why I don't like eating fruits, vegetables, chocolates, chips, this or that, and they keep insisting that I should try whatever they are eating. It is annoying!"

Tonton shouted, trying to let it all out.

"They laugh at me all the time. They call me picky, spoiled, anorexic, and make fun of how my body looks. Today in school the teacher played a video about the importance of eating healthy. Before it played, she said "This is for you, Tonton, since you don't eat anything. Maybe you will learn and will stop being so picky". Everybody laughed. It was terrible, mom. I don't want a party, and I never want to go back to school."

Wiping her tears, Tonton continued: "Why was I born like this, mommy? You always tell me how perfect I am, but I am not. I am different from everyone else, I am weird… I think there is something wrong with me."

"Daddy, I am not a good daughter. I know I make you guys go through a lot; I've noticed how concerned you are that I don't eat like all the other kids."

"I give you a lot of trouble. You don't think I've realized I am the reason we haven't traveled as much or gone to a restaurant recently? That's why I don't want a party anymore. I fear embarrassing myself. I know how much you dreamed of this party for me, I am sorry for letting you down."

"Oh, my love, we don't have to decide anything about your party right now. Just know that the party is not important for me or daddy, you are! And if it means that you will be suffering, then we will cancel it. Don't you worry about it. When I say you are perfect, I mean you are perfect just the way you are. Even with your challenges and difficulties, you are perfect to me and your dad."

In this moment, despite their concern and frustration for having planned something so special for their daughter, Tonton's parents did something extremely important: they did not judge her, they did not punish her, and they validated all the feelings their daughter had expressed. Even if those feelings might not have made sense to them. The fact they were listening to her and trying to empathize with her and making themselves available and open for what she said allowed Tonton to express her emotions.

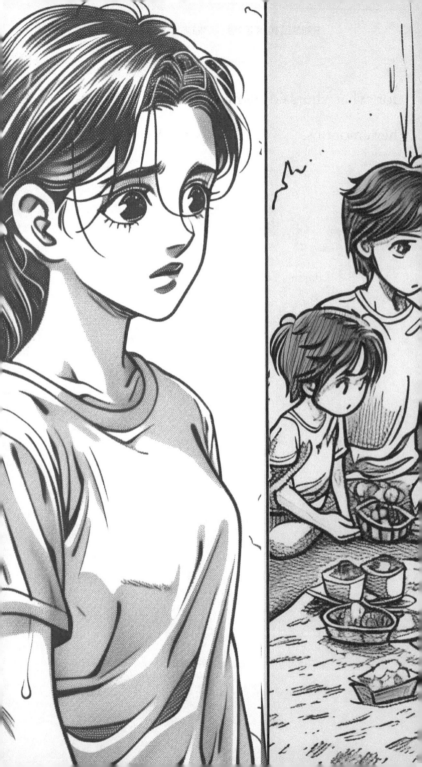

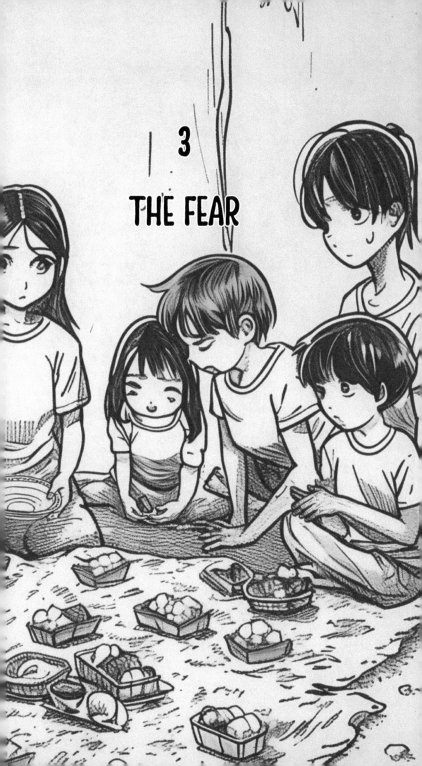

3

THE FEAR

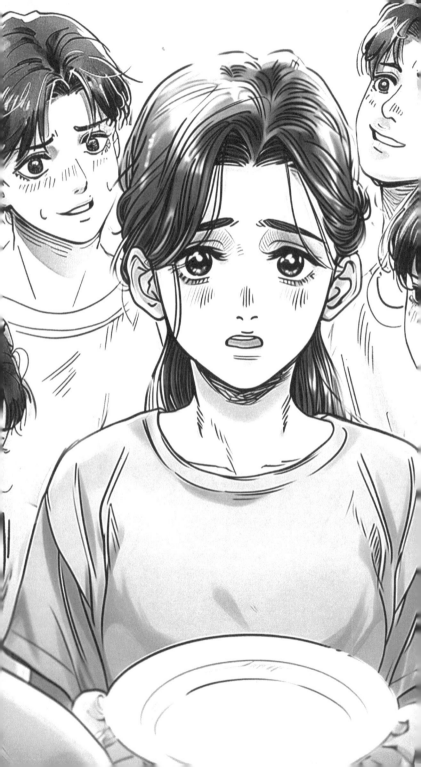

THE FEAR

The fact they were listening to her and trying to empathize with her and making themselves available and open for what she said allowed Tonton to express her emotions.

"So, I don't need to be perfect for you two to love me?"

"Of course not, Tonton. Forgive us if we have not made that clear for you. Forgive us if we have made you think you need to be perfect to be loved." Said Tonton's parents with teary eyes, hugging her daughter tight.Tonton felt accepted and loved by her parents. Now that she was calmer, she continued opening up to her parents:

"You know, when I was younger and people

didn't realize I was so picky to eat, I did not care if all the foods at my party were what everyone enjoyed. Once they started to realize and make fun of me, I noticed that I was different. So, I started to prefer only having what I ate at my parties. This way, I would eat just like everyone else and would not have to deal with people asking me why I didn't like to eat what they thought were the most delicious treats at the party. It is really annoying having to explain and give them excuses. No one understands."

"You remember my birthday party last year here at home? You guys did everything I asked. No finger food, no candies, no hot dogs, no fries. Just popcorn, cheddar goldfish, and vanilla cake."

"You know what Marina said the next day? That at my parties the food isn't too good, all the food I like to eat is no fun. She didn't even bother remembering all the fun games we played and all the fun we had, she just complained that the food wasn't yummy."

"Dad, remember when you asked me why I haven't gone to the school trips recently, or gone to sleepovers at my cousins' and friends' houses?"

"I always had an excuse, but the truth is that I am embarrassed and feel bad for not eating what everyone eats. I feel like everyone keeps staring at me, judging me as if I did it on purpose."

"My friend Ana even said that I do this for attention, but I swear that is not the reason, dad."

"Do you think I would choose to be like this? Embarrassing myself in front of my friends?"

"Why do I not like eating what everyone else does? Why am I so scared to try the things most of my friends eat?"

"I pretended that I wasn't bothered by what my friends said, and even laughed with them when they first started making fun of me. Not anymore, those words hurt me, mom and dad. In those times all I could think of was my room, the only place that made me feel safe."

"Last time I went to Maria's house, her mom said I needed to stay there for a week so that I would learn how to eat right. It seems like people are mad at me all the time. Do I need to eat what people want me to eat for them to be nice to me!? Oh well, I am a failure. I can't even eat right."

"At all my friends' houses, their moms always insist that I eat. I say no to one thing, so they offer me something else, then I say no again, and again… I do get hungry, but if I think about eating those things they offer me… it makes me want to cry! I had to start lying and say that I had eaten at home and wasn't hungry. They would say: "This girl is never hungry, no wonder she is so skinny".

"Everyone always has something to say,

whether it's good or bad. It sucks, I didn't want it to be like this. I swear mom, I swear dad, this is not a choice, I just can't eat like the other kids. I swear I want to be able to."

4

THE DECISION

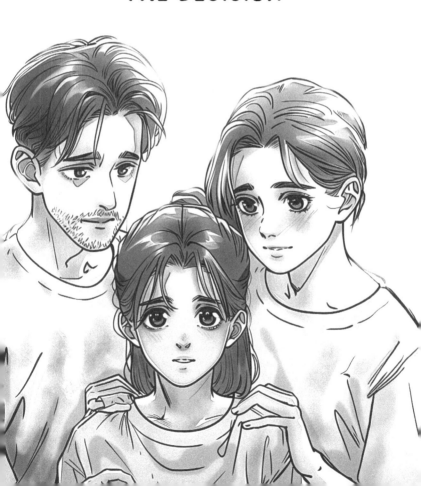

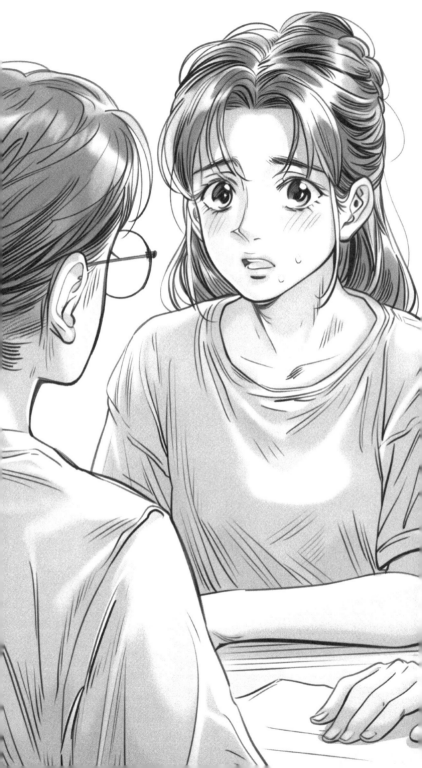

THE DECISION

Until this day, Tonton's parents had no idea how much their daughter was suffering and how they had not noticed how impactful her extreme picky eating was to her social life. It was a very tough moment for them as well.

Ever since Tonton was little, her parents tried to seek help, but they always heard the same thing from all the different professionals:

"It'll pass with time. Your daughter just needs good role models, and she will eat better. The important thing is to never stop offering her food, keep insisting."

"Your daughter needs discipline. Stop spoiling her, all she wants is attention."

"Let her starve, then you will see if she really doesn't eat."

They believed the medical advice and attempted everything they were told.

Without realizing they were only making her eating challenges worse; Tonton's parents pressured her to eat and threatened to ground her. They tried many different strategies, but none of them worked.

Eventually, they gave up. They hoped that with time, as if it were a magic trick, everything would be solved. They started to meet their daughter's needs, bringing her safe foods to restaurants, trips, and friends' houses. They did that until her

FERNANDA DO VALLE AND GIOVANA VASCONCELLOS

safe foods started to narrow down and Tonton did not want to eat if it was not at home. "Time will heal it", they heard. Instead, it only got worse.

After seeing how much Tonton's extreme picky eating was impacting their lives, her parents decided to look for help once again. Now, however, they had more information on their daughter's situation and knew that she wasn't simply being picky. Instead, it was much more serious than that, so they searched for a place that would be understanding of their daughter's difficulties and accommodate for all her needs in this journey.

After a long search, they finally found a place with an incredible team of professionals prepared to help Tonton conquer her fears of eating. A place where they teach kids how to overcome their challenges. It was a "food school" that taught kids how to eat, and as soon as they got there the principal started to explain how everything worked.

"Here, we don't refer to it as "treatment". We call it a learning process. The same way a kid having difficulties with math might need help learning, a kid with eating challenges should also be provided with tutors and private coaches to help them learn and develop skills to eat better."

Tonton loved the comparison, making it easier for her to understand that she was not worse than others due to her difficulties.

The principal went on: "Tonton, we all have our difficulties. We all need help and resources to be able to overcome such difficulties. I'm sure you know someone that needs glasses because they can't see well, or someone that might need help to read. What is happening to you is no one's fault. Not yours, not your parents, no one. It's hard for you to eat certain things because your brain thinks some foods are not safe for you, so it is only trying to protect you."

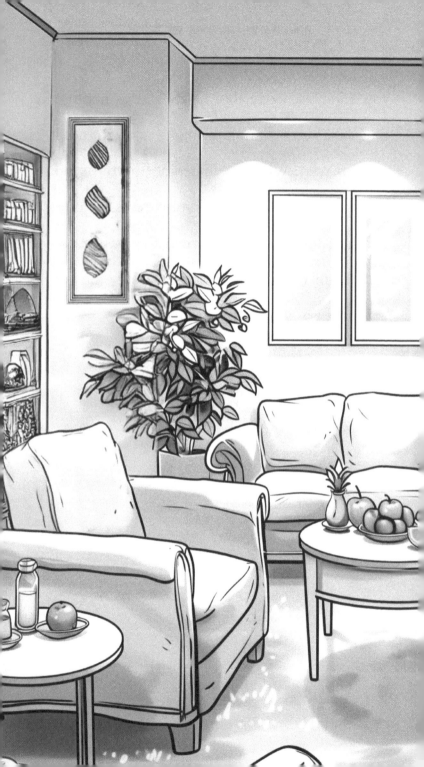

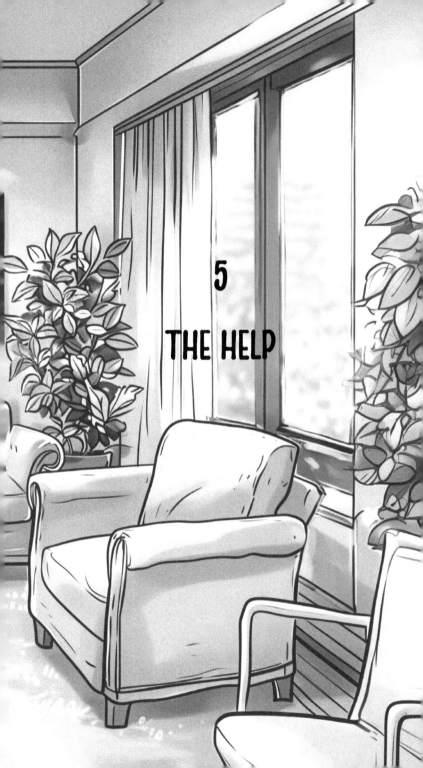

5
THE HELP

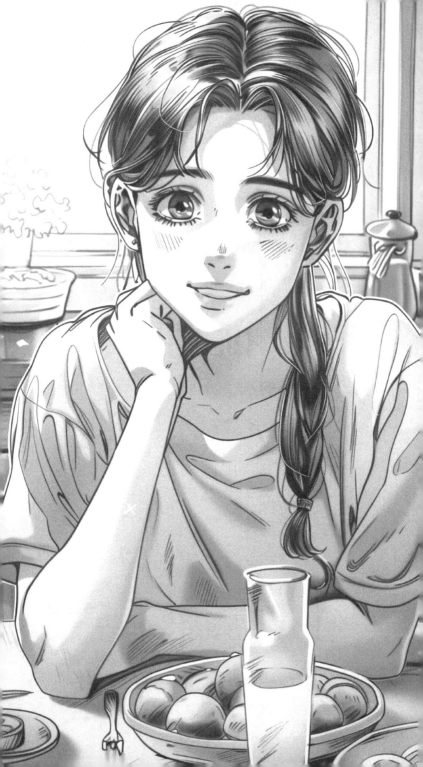

THE HELP

"The good news is that we can teach your brain to understand that you will be safe eating those foods and that it does not need to protect you anymore. With the help of the right people, extreme picky eating can be beaten, and here, you are in the right place with the right people."

"So, I'm not sick?"

"No Tonton, you are not sick. You just need help."

"I am afraid of trying new foods. I'm not even scared; I am frightened of it. I have the desire to try certain things. When I'm in my room by myself, it feels like I have the courage to try something new. I want to be able to eat with my friends, but when the time arrives, for real, I can't do it and I run away."

"I'm afraid I won't be able to swallow correctly, afraid I'll throw up, afraid of what will happen if I try to eat something different. The taste that it will leave in my mouth. I can't even eat a little piece; I don't feel safe. There are some things that I am afraid of, and there are some things that disgust me. Just thinking about it makes me gag and I want to throw up."

"All of these feelings are normal, it's part of your difficulty. Here, we will teach you how to deal with all of this and help you face your fears".

"But how is that possible? I can't put

anything new in my mouth. I just CAN'T! Please don't push me."

"Tonton, we won't do anything until you are ready. Instead of saying "I can't eat this" you will start saying "I am not ready to try this yet", can you do that for me?"

"Yes, I can. So, you won't force me to eat anything?"

"Never. No one will force you to eat. Not here, not at home, nowhere. Eating is the last step of our learning process."

"But if eating is the last step, what am I going to do here?"

"We will explore what foods you are willing to try. You will learn about them, learn to deal with their smell, their texture, and learn how to be near such foods. We will cook them together and have so much fun. It will be something gradual that will take as much time as you need. Each person is unique, so we will plan your learning process according to what works best for you. You are part of this process."

"We will talk about your feelings, your emotions, your fears, and anxieties. You will learn some tricks to deal with the discomfort of feeling scared… It's not about not being scared, Tonton. It's about learning how to face your fears. Not allowing your fears to have control over you, paralyzing you and making you want to run away. You will show your fears that you are the one in control. Just so you know, the fact you are here telling us how you feel is already an act of courage.

It's the first step."

"Together, we will decide which foods we will try first. We will be creating a scale from the easiest to hardest food to try, and step by step we will evolve. At your time, with no pressure."

"I think vegetables will be the hardest."

"That's fine, Tonton. This food group can be challenging for a lot of people. The more you challenge yourself to try them, the easier it gets. You will be surprised with new flavors, and you will start to enjoy foods that you could never have imagined. I guarantee it."

"Wow! I can't wait to come to this school to start learning all of this. I want to be able to live just like all my friends. How long will it take for me to eat better?"

"That depends, Tonton. Remember how I said each person has a different process? I suggest we start the process with foods that will help you return to your social life. What I mean by this is that you will be able to go to a party and eat something, or you will be able to spend the day in school without being hungry. Trying foods that will allow you to sleep over at a friend's house without worrying that you won't like anything they offer you. Foods that will allow you to go to a restaurant with your parents and eat with them, or travel without a "survival kit" with your safe foods, and much more. We don't eat just to nourish our body. We also eat with our friends and our family, and we create memories of what we ate and who we ate with."

"Speaking of friends, Tonton, do you talk about your eating challenges with them?"

"No. I'm embarrassed and scared that no one will like me anymore if they find out who I really am. I told my parents that when my friends started making fun of me, I would laugh with them so that they would still like me. The things they said to me hurt my feelings, so I started to eat by myself and stopped going to my friends' houses so I wouldn't have to eat there. I used to eat more food, but I started to get sick of most of them so now I don't even eat 10 different things. I feel much more comfortable eating the same thing. I feel safer."

"It's normal to start eating less things if you only eat the same food all the time. We will help you with that. What's important is that you stop trying to be someone you are not. Other people must like you just the way you are, with your qualities and flaws. If someone doesn't like you for who you are, that's fine… we don't need everyone to like us. You should never pretend to be someone you aren't just to fit in. The most important thing is that you respect your difficulties and love yourself the way you are. That's how you will be able to overcome your challenges and deal with such a delicate subject to you."

"Tonton, from now on you won't hide your difficulties just for people to like you. Deal?"

"Deal!"

6

PLAN IN ACTION

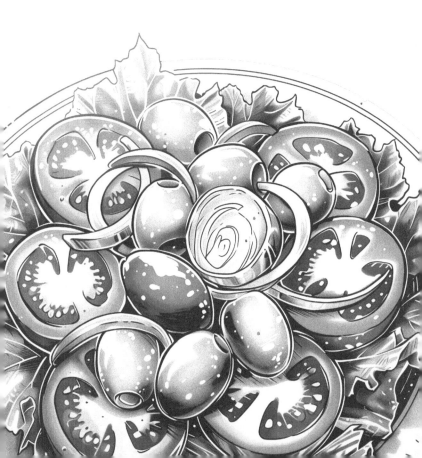

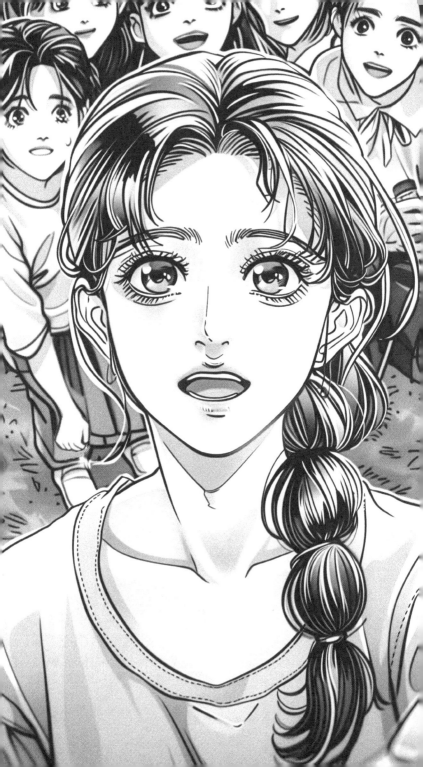

PLAN IN ACTION

Tonton was confident and excited. She still wanted to cancel her 12th birthday party, but she was certain that on her 13th birthday everything would be different.

Tonton's parents were now prepared with a lot of knowledge to help their daughter, and they were relieved to have such a strong support system with capable professionals that respected Tonton the way she was. This time, it seemed like everything was going to work out.

One of the first things they did was talk to Tonton's school about her extreme picky eating, educating them on what they can do to aid Tonton in her process. After all, school is one of the social environments in which kids spend most of their time. It's crucial that the school is open to Tonton's difficulties and that they are involved as facilitators to help her learning process. Her teacher understood the severity of her comments to Tonton before playing the video about healthy eating habits. The teacher recognized her mistake and apologized in front of the whole class. The lack of information causes people to act the wrong way and say things they shouldn't have.

The school learned from what happened and decided to use it as an opportunity to teach all their students about eating difficulties and how important it is to not make any comments on what someone eats or their bodies. We never know what someone is going through and saying something harmful could lead to something even worse, just how it did to Tonton who was isolating herself after what her friends said to her.

Once her friends learned about Tonton's eating challenges, they never made fun of her again and never said anything that could make her feel embarrassed. They understood that many times, even if we are just joking around, we can accidentally "bully" someone, even if that was not our intention. They all learned about empathy and the importance of being careful with what we say, because we can hurt someone we love very deeply.

Tonton told her friends she was going to a "food school" to learn how to eat better, and she was surprised with all the different difficulties each of her friends had to deal with. It was liberating to be able to talk about this in such an open way and to feel seen by people she liked so much.

She saw that she wasn't the only child going through something. Everyone had their own challenges, their own fears, and it was alright if you needed help. In fact, she encouraged many other kids in her school to face their fears. Tonton's fear was of eating, but Marina's was sleeping by herself, Peter was scared no one liked him, John was scared of the dark, and Regina was scared of becoming fat. Renata needs a private math tutor because she has learning difficulties, and Lauren needs help concentrating in class. Jack is horrified that something terrible will happen to his parents, and Joana is terrified of thunder.

Learning about her and her friends' challenges allowed Tonton to see how everyone had their difficulties, and she finally felt like she was part of a group again.

7

THE BIRTHDAY PARTY

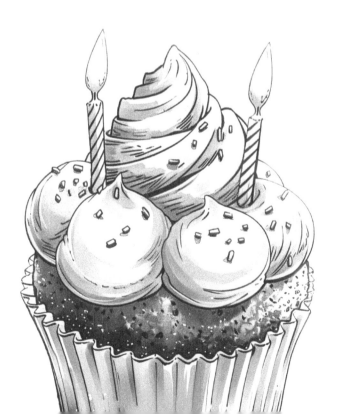

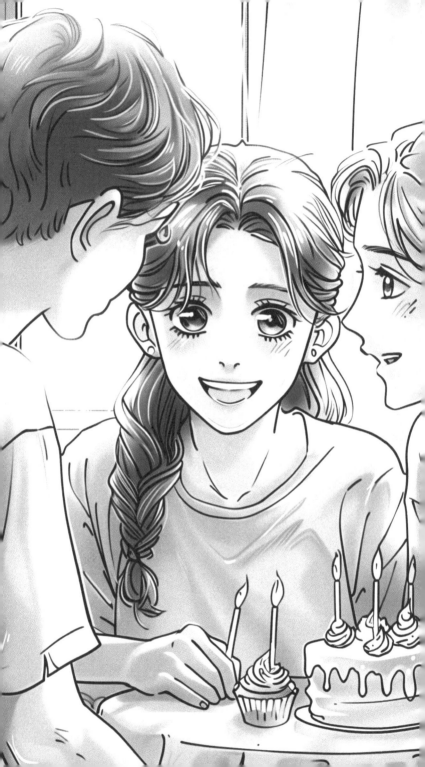

THE BIRTHDAY PARTY

A year later, Tonton celebrated much more than her 13th birthday. She celebrated her courage and how she overcame so many of her challenges. This past year, she went on an adventure, discovering new flavors and creating new memories and stories to tell. She was happy, no longer feeling weird or the need to isolate herself.

She regained her self-esteem and confidence. She made new friendships and learned that she wasn't born to please everyone, what mattered was being herself. Tonton was smiling once again, charming and entertaining everyone around her, just like her old self. This time, however, it was different. She was no longer trying to be someone she wasn't just to be accepted. She stopped being so hard on herself and did not try to hide her difficulties. She no longer tried to be perfect.

The adults learned how essential it was to be accepting of their child's difficulties, and they learned how important it was to be good role models to their children. Never again will they exclude, expose or judge someone for sharing their difficulties.

Tonton not only learned but taught others that perfection does not exist. All of us make mistakes, face challenges, and need help to overcome them.

A WORD TO PARENTS AND CAREGIVERS

Feeding difficulties and eating disorders are not a child's choice, nor are they fussiness or inappropriate behavior to get attention, as many think. Unfortunately, it is not uncommon, even within the medical profession, to find professionals who are not prepared and trained to support these families, blaming the parents or saying that when the child goes to school they will learn to eat, that it's just a phase, that the child is spoiled, among other inappropriate comments. But the good news is that there are specialized treatments, and feeding difficulties can be overcome. If, while reading this book, you identified and realized that your child might have some kind of feeding difficulty, seek help from a specialist in this area.

You are not alone!

Receive our embrace,

Fernanda do Valle

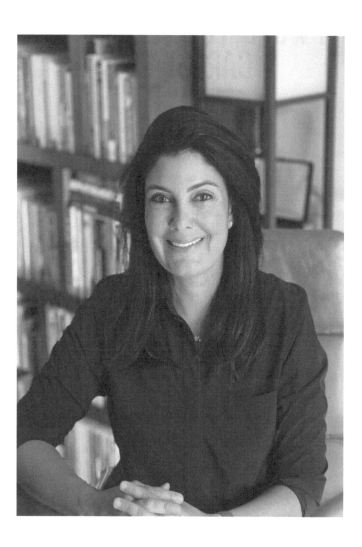

ABOUT THE AUTHORS

Fernanda do Valle was born in Rio de Janeiro, RJ, Brazil on the 17th of March, 1978 and has been a resident in the United States since 2015. She received both her bachelor's and master's degree from Purdue University in Psychology and Applied Behavior Analysis (ABA), respectively. Additionally, Fernanda has a background in neurocoaching, dialectical behavior therapy (DBT), and cognitive behavior therapy in eating disorders (CBT-ED). Ever since recovering from Anorexia Nervosa and consequently publishing her first book "Together: Our Fight Against Anorexia" in 2009, Fernanda has dedicated part of her time giving lectures and has been a source of help for thousands of families through her books and projects which detail both her personal and professional experiences. The author is the mother of Daniel and Theo (the source of inspiration for her book "ARFID (Avoidant Restrictive Food Intake Disorder): A Guide for Parents and Caregivers", in which she shares her son's extreme picky eating and their arduous journey in search of the cure).

"It was due to the lack of specialists who could help my son that I became one!", said Fernanda do Valle.

Fernanda has published eight books in Brazil, two of which have been translated to English by Underline Publishing. The author is also a member of the International Academy of Brazilian Literature, who have awarded her the prize of International Recognition of Brazilian Literature in 2020 and 2023 in New York.

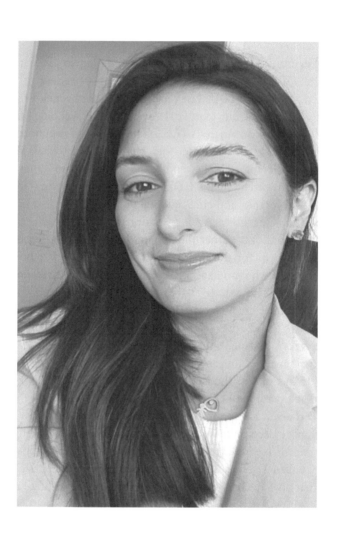

Giovana Vasconcellos was born on the 18th of January, 1990 in Campinas, SP, Brazil and graduated from PUC (Campinas, SP, Brazil) in psychology with a focus in Behavior Analysis. Giovana has more than 10 years of experience with Applied Behavior Analysis (ABA), working directly with the development of children on the Autism Spectrum, and has practiced as an ABA therapist, an ABA supervisor, and an administrator of clinical cases. She has a Master of Business Administration (MBA) in leadership, management, and productivity. Since adolescence, Giovana knew her focus would be in working with children, aiding and participating in their development as a whole. She is the mother of Antonella, who inspired the author to share her knowledge of stimulus and child development with families, caretakers and professionals.

"Ever since I became a mom, I have noticed a great imposition of rules to achieve perfect child development. Combining my technical knowledge with my maternal experience, I reinforced my idea that we must consider familial contexts and each child unique to each case to successfully monitor development. That is why I began my journey of sharing my knowledge and real-life experiences, in which it was not always possible to apply what was ideal, but instead what was possible," said Giovana Vasconcellos.

Made in United States
Troutdale, OR
09/12/2024

22759896R00040